MW00452144

EVADING EBOLA

Decrease Your Risk of Infection, Fare Far Better If Exposed

David DeRose, MD, MPH

COMPASSHEALTH CONSULTING, INC.
FORESTHILL, CALIFORNIA

Copyright © 2014 by CompassHealth Consulting, Inc.

Published in the United States of America

All Rights Reserved

Edited by Ken McFarland, Page One Communications

Cover Design by Vikiana Pinova

Publisher's Notice

Reproduction in whole or part of this publication without express written consent is strictly prohibited. The author greatly appreciates the time you're investing to improve your health by reading this book. Please help extend the influence of this important topic by leaving a review where you bought the book, or telling your friends about it. Thank you.

The information in this book is designed for educational purposes only. It is not intended to be a substitute for informed medical advice or care. You should not use the information provided to diagnose or treat any health problems or illnesses without first consulting your primary health care giver.

ISBN: 978-0-9743990-8-9

Contents

About the Author

Heard on more than 140 radio stations, syndicated radio show host and practicing physician, David DeRose, MD, MPH, has been helping people address disease processes with natural therapies for some three decades. DeRose brings solid credentials as a board-certified specialist in both Internal Medicine and Preventive Medicine, in addition to holding a Masters in Public Health degree with an emphasis in Health Promotion and Health Education. DeRose's research has been published in peer-reviewed medical journals, including the *Journal of the American Medical Association*, the *Annals of Epidemiology*, and *Preventive Medicine*.

Known for his engaging and practical presentations, Dr. DeRose will keep you on the edge of your seat with skills honed as an award-winning public speaker, published medical researcher, syndicated talk radio host, and college teacher.

Dedication

To Sonja, for her undying affection and support.

Foreword

In reflecting on my Internal Medicine training, two key principles stand out in my mind regarding the management of medical emergencies and other crises. The first, articulated by a famous American of yesteryear, is this: ***Don't just stand there—do something***. The second is similar to the first, yet, radically different: ***Don't just do something—stand there***.

As the world faces a potential global Ebola pandemic, these two important principles strike me as increasingly relevant. The first reminds us that when the time comes to act, we must act with alacrity and efficiency. Already, the U.S. response to the crisis has revealed gaps in this first principle.

However, the second principle is equally important. No value lies in doing, merely to be doing something. At each step in our response, individually and societally, we need to have well-thought-out reasons supporting our strategies and tactics.

The American public—and lay people throughout the Western World—need to do both. With this in mind, this book lays out a simple three-step approach:

▶ First, we need to be clear on essential aspects of Ebola—some of which have so far eluded the lay press. Foremost, as I explain in the first chapter, you can have a major exposure to Ebola and not contract the disease.

▶ Second, as I spend most of this book explaining, despite our limitations in Ebola knowledge, the history of virology has given us some powerful insights into how to protect ourselves from killer viruses. Applying these insights could well make the difference between life and death.

▸ Third, only when we understand the fundamentals of the virus—and approaches we can all employ to decrease our risk—are we really ready to do something.

So—*just stand here* with me in the pages of this book—long enough to understand key practical principles of Ebola prevention. Then *do something*: Apply those principles on a daily basis. With such a game plan, I believe that most of us, even if exposed, can evade Ebola.

—David DeRose, MD, MPH
Foresthill, CA, November 13, 2014

Introduction

Intense media coverage has ensured that most of us have already been asking "Ebola questions."

- ▸ What happens if I'm exposed?
- ▸ How can I decrease my risk?
- ▸ What should our country—and our communities—be doing?

Such questions are especially relevant to health professionals. After all, at least in Western nations, we currently stand at probably the highest risk of acquiring this highly lethal infection.

From the standpoint of Ebola, some would say I'm fortunate. Although a board-certified Internal Medicine specialist, I'm currently doing relatively little in the clinical realm. (Last year I scaled back my Internal Medicine practice to devote more time to CompassHealth Consulting, Inc.—the consulting and media company I have operated for the past dozen years.) Nonetheless, I still see patients sporadically. Despite my limited patient contact, I still found myself asking the question: What would I do if I learned I had been exposed to a patient with Ebola?

Let's make the scenario more poignant. I become exposed to the virus during a physical exam when a patient (with no foreign travel history and no obvious history of Ebola exposure) vomits on me—before anyone realizes she actually has the disease. In other words, I hadn't donned any protective gear—and I have a significant exposure. Am I doomed to sit in quarantine until I come down with the dreaded infection?

The evidence, fortuitously, says no. (Not to the advisability of quarantine but rather to the certainty of my acquiring a clinical—or overt—infection with Ebola.) As I explain in the next chapter, the first piece of good news about Ebola is indeed this: Even following a significant exposure to the virus, contracting the disease is not inevitable.

But there's more good news. As I spend most of this book explaining, despite our limited knowledge of Ebola, medical science has provided powerful insights into how to protect ourselves from killer infections. I'll walk you through eight key strategies calculated to help you avoid ever becoming infected with Ebola—and if you are exposed—to decrease your risk of infection.

Granted, the multi-step approach I'm promoting has not been **proven** to make humans Ebola-proof. But I'm convinced it has the potential to significantly decrease your risk of this modern plague. Furthermore, by applying the principles in this book, you'll actually help answer one of today's most pressing questions: How can I decrease my risk of Ebola once exposed?

Why am I so confident? This book is not the collections of a rambling physician who has a passion for flipping coins. As you'll learn in chapter 3, nearly two decades ago I teamed up with other researchers to help address another international epidemic: diabetes and its complication of nerve damage (neuropathy). We used the same four-step theoretical approach I'm outlining in this book:

1. Look at promising, even if unproven, natural strategies in the literature.

2. Share the information with patients.

3. Compare the outcomes of those who follow selected strategies with those who don't.

4. Draw conclusions.

In that research, ultimately presented at the largest annual gathering of public health and preventive medicine experts in the world (the 1990 annual session of the American Public Health Association), we demonstrated several things. First, diabetic patients could improve nerve symptoms by 20 percent to 45 percent in a few weeks. Second, a number (but not all) of the simple natural strategies we recommended were associated with improvement.

The lesson for Ebola is simple. Research suggests we can do a number of simple things to help stop the spread of the disease. I can't conclusively say that every one of my strategies will ultimately be proven to make a difference. However, I'm confident the formula can render most of us able, even if exposed, to evade Ebola.

CHAPTER ONE

Good News About Ebola

Recently, I asked Edna, my 96-year-old mother-in-law, "Mama, did you know you had polio when you were little?" She quickly countered, "I never had polio." Actually, we probably were both right.

To a layperson, my assessment of our brief conversation likely sounds nonsensical. Most would reason that a person either had or didn't have polio—there's no way she could be in both categories. However, things are not quite so simple.

Polio, like many other viruses, can cause something called an "inapparent infection." In such cases a person does indeed become infected with the virus, but they never develop the expected clinical illness. In Edna's case, I was speculating that she was indeed exposed to the polio virus but never had the severe nerve and muscle involvement that goes along with a full-blown case of the disease. In fact, in the era before vaccination for poliomyelitis (the full name of the condition) there is evidence to suggest far more people were exposed to the virus—and fought it off—than those who succumbed to the illness.

The same is true of many other potentially lethal viruses. Every year thousands of Americans come down with influenza—and don't even know it. Their illness is so mild that they either feel fine, or perhaps experience a bit more fatigue for a couple of days. Antibody testing, however, doesn't lie—they were exposed to the flu virus, and their immune systems fought it off.

Have you ever heard of "equine encephalitis"? This family of brain-infecting viruses can affect humans as well as horses. Human infection can cause death or permanent brain disability. However, the vast majority of people infected with these viruses never realize they were exposed. Their inapparent infection went undetected.

What about Ebola? Is there any evidence of inapparent infection with this lethal disease? Most definitely. Despite the paucity of media reporting on this important topic, the evidence has been clear for well over a decade: Many of those exposed to Ebola never get sick with the disease.

In 1996 Ebola reared its ugly head in the African nation of Gabon. The particular strain—the serotype—was the same one involved in the 2014 epidemic; namely, the Zaire variety. (I'll talk more about the basics of Ebola infection in the next chapter.) Not unexpectedly, the disease claimed the lives of some 70 percent of those who came down with clinical illness.

However, an astute team of Gabonese physicians made a remarkable discovery. They identified twenty-four close contacts of patients. Each had been "directly exposed to infected materials" (either feces, vomit, saliva, sweat, or blood). Nevertheless, not one of the twenty-four ever became ill. Perhaps even more remarkably, as reported by Eric Leroy and colleagues in the British journal, *The Lancet*, blood testing revealed that eleven of the twenty-four showed they had become infected with the Ebola virus, *yet never became sick.*

The paper is encouraging for at least two reasons. First, you can be in close proximity to Ebola with not a scrap of protective gear, be exposed to infective secretions, and never become infected (as occurred with thirteen of the twenty-four in the study just cited). But second, even if the Ebola virus gets a foothold in your body, you have the potential to fight it off without ever getting sick.

Although the researchers apparently never performed an epidemiologic study in an attempt to identify modifiable factors that may have helped protect these two dozen individuals, the Gabonese team did discover something of relevance in their earlier work: "We have found that immunological events very early in an Ebola-virus infection determine the control of viral replication and recovery or catastrophic illness and death." The implications are clear: A person's immune status at the time of, and shortly following, Ebola virus exposure is a key factor, making the difference between life and death.

In other words, there is no direct, beaten path from Ebola exposure to quarantine to infection and finally to death. We can be exposed to Ebola-infected secretions and not become infected ourselves. Furthermore, if infected with the Ebola virus, we don't have to get sick.

Consequently, when dealing with Ebola, our focus needs to be four-fold:

▶ Do all we can to avoid or limit our exposure to the virus. But if exposed (or potentially exposed) apply the following three strategies:

▶ Enhance our immune status in general.

▶ Improve our immune system's antiviral capacities.

▶ Employ techniques to decrease viral survivability.

Although our understanding is still incomplete when it comes to the best ways to address Ebola per se, the science of virology reveals a number of factors that can make a profound difference between succumbing to infection and eradicating even a "killer virus." Likely, a number of these strategies will give you the upper hand in dealing with Ebola.

Yes, the message is clear: We can likely evade Ebola's tentacles. In the next chapter, we'll take a look at the science behind Ebola infection and then launch into a host of potentially life-saving strategies.

CHAPTER TWO

A Brief Ebola Primer

Viruses, simply put, are packets of infectious genetic material (either RNA or DNA) which lack the ability to replicate without a living host. Once a virus infects an organism, it can insert its RNA or DNA into host cells and orchestrate a mass production process that replicates itself.

We have a number of lines of defense against viral illness, including such mundane topics as avoidance and preserving intact skin. However, once infected, you rely on your immune system to eradicate the foreign invaders.

In order to best plan our approach to evading Ebola, we need to know more than viral generalities. We need to look more closely at the enemy. Let's take a quick survey with that in mind.

The Ebola virus was first identified in 1976 in the context of an outbreak affecting over 300 people in Northern Zaire, Africa. (The virus traces its moniker to this first outbreak, which occurred in the vicinity of the Ebola River.) Although details can be difficult to piece together after an event, one likely scenario describing the outbreak follows.

The index case (the first person connected to the disease) appeared to have contracted Ebola while working in a rat-

and bat-infested cotton factory in Nzara, Sudan. After several days he arrived at a local hospital for treatment. Apparently he was presumptively treated for malaria, receiving a chloroquine malaria shot under unfortunate infection-control circumstances. (It was ultimately discovered that the hospital was reusing needles without adequate sterilization.) The infection was then spread to other hospital patients who received "treatment" with the same, now-infected needle. Soon the infection spread to hospital workers and others in the community.

Family Matters

The Ebola virus and the related Marburg virus are the only two known members of the filovirus family (*Filoviridae* in Latin). The family name is derived from the fact that microscopically, these viruses can be seen to be strand-like filaments. Whereas only one species of Marburg virus exists, there are five recognized Ebola species or subtypes. Each of the Ebola variants presents distinctive levels of risk when it comes to human infection. *Zaire Ebola virus,* implicated in that first 1976 outbreak as well as the current 2014 epidemic, is generally regarded as the most lethal once clinical infection develops. Three other species are found in Africa—*Sudan Ebola virus, Taï Forest Ebola virus* (formerly known as Ivory Coast or Côte d'Ivoire Ebola virus) and *Bundibugyo Ebola virus.* The fifth Ebola species, known as *Reston Ebola virus,* has been found to reside exclusively in the Philippines. Reston so far has not been documented to cause human illness. Clinical infections have been limited to non-human primates and pigs.

Ebola Fundamentals

When it comes to Ebola's infectivity, there is much we know—and much still in question. However, the majority of what the lay media has presented squares with the evidence. This includes the following:

▸ Ebola virus is likely maintained in African animal populations such as bats, which apparently often do not succumb to the disease. The disease is sporadically introduced into humans by eating infected animals ("bushmeat") or through direct contact with dead infected animals.

▸ Once a single human case arises, the virus is often spread by human-to-human transmission. (However, historically, some "outbreaks" have involved only an index case; i.e., a single person, with no transmission to other humans.)

▸ Ebola virus appears to be very difficult to transmit prior to clinical illness (i.e., prior to a person having demonstrable evidence of disease). Consequently, it seems extremely unlikely that an entirely asymptomatic individual could transmit the virus—especially through casual contact.

▸ The incubation period for Ebola—the time it takes from exposure to development of symptoms—can range from 2 to 21 days. The average incubation period is between 8 and 10 days.

▸ When a person is clinically infected with Ebola, virus levels in the body increase exponentially during the early course of clinical illness. Compared to the asymptomatic state, viral levels are typically 1,000-fold higher two days into clinical illness and 10,000-fold when they reach their peak on the third to fifth day of symptoms. As a result, a person showing signs and symptoms of Ebola, such as fever, severe headache, sore throat, muscle pains, abdominal pain, diarrhea, vomiting, and bleeding or bruising should be assumed to be highly infectious.

▸ Although Ebola is a cause of what is called viral

hemorrhagic fever, visible bleeding is not typically present—at least early in the course of the illness. If a person's immune system neutralizes the infection early on, she may avoid any of the coagulation defects which accompany severe Ebola illness.

▸ Among Ebola-infected patients, the most infectious body fluids are blood, feces, and vomit. The bodies of those who have recently died from Ebola are also highly infectious. Breast milk, saliva, tears, urine, semen, and the skin (possibly sweat) may also contain the virus. Of note here is the persistence of virus in semen. Men who have contracted Ebola but recovered might be able to transmit the virus through semen for three months or perhaps slightly longer. Therefore, men who have recovered from Ebola are advised either to abstain from sex or to use condoms for at least three months.

▸ Once exposed to the virus a person can become infected by either ingesting the virus (eating without washing one's contaminated hands) or introducing it to his mucous membranes (by rubbing one's eyes or nose). The Ebola virus can also enter the body through breaks in the skin.

Other details about Ebola have not been widely circulated. However, an understanding of these points can also aid us in decreasing our risk of exposure:

▸ Because we only have a limited experience with Ebola, some wonder if some individuals may ultimately demonstrate a longer incubation period than 21 days. This seems possible, but unlikely. However, there is a practical application: the 21-day mark is not a magic number. If you are reading this book following an Ebola exposure, I would recommend you consider continuing the immune-enhancing strategies in this book for at least 28 days from your last date of exposure.

▸ Ebola affects people across the age range. Previous epidemics have affected everyone from neonates to the elderly—and every age category in between. This is an extremely important piece of data as far as the approach I'm advocating in this book.

Here's why: Certain lethal viruses are actually more harmful to those in the prime of health. Such was the case of the Spanish Flu of 1918 and the more recent Hanta virus that surfaced in the Four Corners area of the U.S. Southwest. Both of these viral illnesses seemed most devastating to those with strong immune systems. Immune over-reaction seemed to be one of the main preconditions for fatality. Consequently, the very young and the very old were often spared the most devastating consequences of these diseases.

Although there is evidence of immune system over-reaction in advanced Ebola infection, the evidence indicates that a strong immune system can prevent Ebola from ever getting a strong foothold, thus keeping the infection at bay. Clearly, when it comes to Ebola, an optimally functioning immune system is an asset, not a liability.

Airborne Ebola?

Much controversy has centered on whether Ebola virus could be airborne. I believe public health officials have properly tried to allay anxiety about this route of transmission. The evidence suggests that such airborne exposure is extremely unlikely. However, none of the experts believe such transmission is impossible (in contrast to the messaging sometimes coming through lay channels). The CDC summarized the state of the science well: "Airborne transmission of Ebola virus has been hypothesized but not demonstrated in humans. While Ebola virus can be spread through airborne particles under experimental conditions in animals, this type of spread has not been documented during human EVD outbreaks in settings such as hospitals or households." Furthermore, they acknowledge specifically that previous outbreak investigations have identified Ebola patients who had no known direct contact with other infected individuals, "leading to speculation regarding transmission via aerosolized virus particles."

However, remember this: Unless you are a health care professional, you aren't likely to come into close proximity to anyone shedding Ebola virus in their respiratory secretions. Furthermore, because Ebola does not typically involve coughing or sneezing, this route of transmission is rendered even more unlikely. Nonetheless, this possibility does explain one thing: Those being most careful in dealing with infected patients may, from an abundance of caution, wear "space suits" that obviate the possibility of respiratory droplets being inhaled or landing on exposed areas of skin.

For at least one simple reason this is worth emphasizing for the benefit of health professionals. You see, standard "droplet precautions" are designed to protect individuals from infectious agents that are primarily communicated by the respiratory/mucous membrane routes. With this in mind, a gown, face mask, eye protection, and gloves are typically all that is deemed necessary. However, due to Ebola's ability to enter the body through a variety of routes (including ingestion and through breaks in the skin), the possibility of aerosolized infectious matter makes the case for covering all skin surfaces. Having said this, in hot and humid developing world conditions, where air conditioning is often lacking, other considerations may win out. Maximal personal protective equipment, even if available, could subject caregivers to excessive heat stress, which might outweigh the small theoretical risk of airborne exposure to the virus.

Dogs and Other Sources of Ebola Exposure?

The lay public has become concerned about how the companion animals of Ebola-infected patients have been handled. Why would a dog be euthanized or quarantined just because it lived in the home of an Ebola patient?

The answer probably resides with a fascinating African study published in 2005 in the medical journal *Emerging Infectious Diseases*. There, Loïs Allela and colleagues from Gabon, Africa, studied over 400 dogs for immune evidence of Ebola infection. When they limited their analysis to villages that had both Ebola human cases and documented infected animal carcasses, over 30 percent of pet dogs showed blood evidence of past Ebola infection. None were ever clinically ill. The infected dogs likely contracted Ebola by eating carcasses of other animals that had succumbed to the disease. However, acquiring Ebola from a source patient could not be excluded (by licking up vomitus or other body fluids, for example). The bottom line—and public health concern—is that dogs can have inapparent infections. They can thus be a source of introducing Ebola or perpetuating Ebola in a region.

Ebola exposure can also occur through inanimate objects. Called "fomites" in medical circles, articles used or handled by Ebola patients can carry infectious virus particles. In previous Ebola outbreaks, at least one case was traced to a blanket that had been used by an infected individual. Other studies of blankets used by individuals with Ebola were unable to demonstrate viral contamination. The messages that emerge from this evidence are three-fold:

First, there probably is a small risk of transmission from clothing, bedding, etc. used by those with clinical illness.

Second, most experts would consider the risk of fomite transmission from patients with pre-clinical Ebola infection to be so small as to preclude any significant risk. For this reason, no special precautions are being taken when it comes to inanimate objects such as airplane seats and unsoiled bathroom door handles.

Third, because the possibility of fomite transmission is not zero, if the scope of the epidemic expands in the U.S., or in another region where you find yourself, I would act as if all surfaces could potentially be contaminated. Recommendations in view of this are found in chapter 4.

Summary

The media and expert groups have been providing us with much excellent information about the Ebola virus. However, some lesser-known facts plead for our attention. A more comprehensive understanding of Ebola underscores the case for all of us doing what we can to improve our immune status in the face of the current outbreak.

Perhaps more than this, although many in the political and public health arenas alike seem to think reassurance is critical at this point, I beg to differ. Attempts to minimize the risks of Ebola have largely backfired, as some of those assurances have proved vapid. No, I'm not trying to feed mass hysteria. But I think we've been too worried about such a scenario. Instead, we need to be encouraging Americans—and the denizens of Western nations in general—to live an *Ebola-Aware Lifestyle*.

That's right—"Ebola Aware." As I point out in the chapters that follow, such a lifestyle neither paralyzes us with fear—nor confines us to Hazmat suits in our bedrooms. Rather, it is a lifestyle that recognizes today we all face some finite risk of Ebola exposure, yet realizes we can be proactive about it. We can actually make lifestyle choices that help us evade Ebola, even in the current milieu.

CHAPTER THREE

An Ebola-Evading Game Plan

In the 1990s, while at the Lifestyle Center of America, Dr. Zeno Charles-Marcel and I were seeing a large number of patients who were suffering from severe nerve problems related to diabetes. The medical diagnosis was "distal symmetric diabetic polyneuropathy." For example, one gentleman had such severe pain that he had to quit his white collar job. Another was so affected that he could barely sleep.

At the time, we were applying a host of lifestyle and other natural therapies to help improve diabetes and other chronic diseases. We were already seeing patients make significant improvement with these non-drug approaches. However, we wanted to take things one step farther. Based on our review of the medical literature, we found evidence suggesting a number of natural therapies could provide additional benefits for diabetic nerve problems.

We consequently began combing the medical literature on a quest for dietary supplements that might help diabetic nerves. We identified some eight or ten of them. Over the next several months we carefully monitored the next thirty patients who came to our clinic with severe diabetic neuropathy. Each one was given a summary of the supplements that had shown some preliminary evidence of benefiting their nerve condition. The patients were then at liberty to choose which, if any, of these agents they wanted to add to their regimen. Diabetic neuropathy symptoms were recorded at the time of their first visit and then two to three weeks later.

After all the data was collected, we carefully analyzed the evidence in conjunction with Loma Linda University. When the analysis was complete, we found an average of roughly 20 percent improvement in diabetic neuropathy symptoms (things such as burning, pain, and pins-and-needles sensations)—even when individuals used none of the supplements. This was presumably due to other components of the comprehensive program. However, what was really amazing was this: The use of four specific supplements was associated with significantly greater improvement—around 50 percent on average. (If you're interested, those supplements were alpha lipoic acid, myo-inositol, gamma linolenic acid, and vitamin E.) The other supplements afforded no obvious benefits. None emerged as harmful.

Applying a Similar Strategy to Ebola

The Ebola prevention program I map out in the following pages is not driven by dietary supplements. However, the philosophy is the same as the one that guided our diabetes research nearly two decades ago. Namely, look at all the promising simple strategies available. Then, give people an opportunity to choose which of those agencies to employ. Finally, if a pocket of Ebola infection surfaces in an area, compare those who followed the recommended practices with those who didn't. This will allow us to validate whether or not the remedies in question were truly efficacious.

Let's consider this approach in the context of a hypothetical example. Matilda, a 90-year-old African woman comes from Liberia to the United States. She is appropriately screened at each of the initial steps in her journey, as she first boards a plane at Roberts International Airport in Liberia, connects in Lagos, Nigeria, and then travels on to London's Heathrow Airport. At each of those airports Matilda is carefully questioned regarding Ebola. She recalls no exposures in Liberia, feels fine, and is found to have a normal body temperature.

By the time she clears customs in New York, Matilda is feeling weak and tired (granted, she's been traveling for over twenty-four hours at this point). Additionally, her stomach is upset, but she attributes it to the strange food and beverages on the plane. She says nothing about her "mild" abdominal symptoms to the customs agent. Since Matilda is still afebrile (not feverish), she is allowed to board a flight to Los Angeles for the final leg of her trip.

While on the flight to LAX, the plane runs into a lot of turbulence. Not familiar with the drill, Matilda fails to search for one of those ubiquitous "barf bags" when her stomach becomes even more agitated. Instead, she tries to make it to the bathroom. As she's struggling to get out of her window seat, oblivious to the flight attendant's cries to heed the "Fasten Seat Belt" sign, she finally loses her stomach contents. I'll spare you further details regarding the incident. However, suffice it to say a number of her fellow passengers are exposed to Matilda's body fluids.

As the suddenly alarmed flight crew pieces together her travel history, they radio ahead for a medical team. Those passengers not yet aware of what transpired in the back of the plane are further agitated by the "space suited" health care providers who greet the plane and the public health response that follows. The worst news comes the next day. An afebrile Matilda is diagnosed with Ebola.

No doubt that hypothetical scenario evoked many questions and reactions. Some, I'll answer momentarily. However, the main reason for the scenario is this: If you were exposed to Ebola-laden secretions on that plane with Matilda but were following the recommendations in this book at the time, I'm willing to hazard a highly educated guess. Namely, you'll be less likely to come down with a clinical Ebola infection than someone else on that plane, similarly exposed but not following the recommendations in the ensuing chapters.

Furthermore, once the epidemiologic investigation of Matilda's contacts has been completed, I would hope the investigators would look closely at all I've recommended in this book. I think we'll find a number of the practices outlined here will be connected with protection from Ebola virus clinical disease.

Beyond Conjecture

Some no doubt will criticize my hypothetical scenario. They will argue that current public health measures would preclude such a major exposure to Ebola. I'm not convinced. Nonetheless, we have evidence from previous Ebola outbreaks that is beyond conjecture. Specifically, many people will become exposed to the virus—and will have no idea of the source of their exposure. This was graphically illustrated following a 1995 outbreak of Ebola in Kikwit, Democratic Republic of Congo. A collaborative research team comprised of CDC experts as well as European investigators did extensive blood screening in order to determine evidence of past Ebola infection in Kikwit and surrounding villages. Perhaps the most notable finding was this: nearly 10 percent of villagers examined (15 of 161) showed evidence of past Ebola infection. However, none of these had ever evidenced clinical Ebola infection—none even had a family member who did. Furthermore, only a third (5 of the 15) even knew of a friend or acquaintance with Ebola.

Two messages emerge. First, whether you're on a flight with Matilda, or it's a bathroom door handle or some bills exchanged at your local grocery store, if Ebola is rampant in a region, you run significant risk of virus exposure. But second, remember, all of these people were survivors—and none had clinical illness. This book is written to help you decrease your exposure. However, even if you're exposed, I'm determined to do all I can to help you not only live to tell about it—but to do so without ever becoming ostensibly ill with Ebola.

But What About Those Unanswered Questions?

I realize there is some risk in framing that airplane nightmare featuring Matilda. I'm not trying to further stoke Ebola fears, but the hypothetical account adds some important points to the Ebola dialogue.

No doubt, many of you are wondering how someone could have Ebola infection and yet have no fever. I'll be the first to admit I'm not an Ebola specialist; however, I do have formal training in Infectious Disease medicine by virtue of my Internal Medicine background, as well as epidemiology and outbreak investigation experience through my Public Health/ Preventive Medicine training.

What we know in the general field of communicable infectious diseases is straightforward: Many illnesses that normally produce a fever may not do so in an immunocompromised host. Such individuals may be on immune-suppressing drugs for autoimmune disease or following an organ transplant. Or they may have a weaker immune system due to extremes of age (either very young or very old). Although I have not seen definitive data making the connection between immune deficiencies and presenting with no fever in the face of early Ebola infection, I would not be surprised if such is the case. We do know unequivocally that more than 10 percent of patients during the current West African outbreak had no elevation in temperature from the time symptoms began to the time they were diagnosed at a medical facility.

Let me attempt both to allay some anxiety as well as to make a case for being serious about one premise of this book. Specifically, ensuring we are following a lifestyle that optimizes our immune systems may be one of our best lines of protection if exposed to Ebola.

If Matilda had been carefully evaluated using the CDC's current algorithm and checklist, she likely would not have been allowed to board the LAX flight. (See http://www.cdc.gov/vhf/ebola/pdf/ebola-algorithm.pdf; http://www.cdc.gov/vhf/ebola/pdf/checklist-patients-evaluated-us-evd.pdf).

However, let's face it: Screeners are still getting used to these new protocols—and some people may slip through the cracks. Furthermore, no matter how effective the person doing the screening, in the absence of fever or other identifiable signs of illness, we're forced to rely on the integrity of the traveler.

The reality is this: It's no different in Africa than America. Many of us will try to deny we're ill until forced to admit we have a problem. If you don't believe me, just sit in the waiting room of a hospital's emergency department. Of course, it wouldn't be appropriate to ask each person who came through the doors how long they had symptoms before showing up there. However, if you could follow one of the E.D. physicians, it would shock you the number of people who attributed their heart-related chest pain to indigestion, the bleeding from their colon cancer to "hemorrhoids," and their brain hemorrhage-related headache to "just a migraine." You get the picture.

Such a realization might temper our judgment of someone like Matilda minimizing his or her symptoms. But should we? Just because we tend to downplay our own symptoms, should there be any excuse for a person from an Ebola-stricken region to dismiss early signs of infection? After all, we're not only talking a personal health threat—but a serious public health issue.

Should We Ban All Flights From West Africa?

I tend to side with most public health experts who feel this would be a mistake. Yet I won't be dogmatic. If you're in the camp arguing for further travel restrictions, I respect your desire to do what you believe would decrease our risk in this nation. I won't discuss this at length here, because it really is a tangential issue to the main points in this book. However, let me share just two reasons why I believe further travel restrictions may well be misguided.

First, borders tend to be porous overseas. I believe the concerns are legitimate that restricting access to the U.S. from certain regions might only incentivize circumvention of those restrictions. Such attempts are likely to include deception with its corollary of failing to get prompt evaluation for Ebola symptoms. In other words, a more open policy where we attempt to win the confidence of those coming within our borders may do more to help with early detection and treatment of foreign travelers. After all, it's undetected and/or untreated illness that poses the greatest threat.

Second, the ultimate mitigation of Ebola risk in America will only come when the current epidemic is quelled in West Africa. If Americans are going to significantly impact that raging Ebola epidemic overseas we likely will need more than the U.S. military, the CDC, and other governmental agencies. From the outset, some of the front line efforts by Westerners have been coordinated under the auspices of nongovernmental organizations (NGOs). The first two Americans sickened by Ebola—Nancy Writebol and Kent Brantly—were among that number. Some of these NGOs historically have been very effective at marshaling short-term volunteer health workers to serve in stricken regions. To enact travel bans would essentially close doors to some sources of needed medical assistance. (For example, a doctor who might be willing to help in Guinea during her two-week vacation would not likely venture out of the U.S. if she couldn't fly back home.)

The bottom line is this: the Ebola virus is now on American soil. I'm in favor of doing all we can to decrease our risk of further source patients, but my emphasis in this chapter is simple. No matter what we do, it is likely—until the epidemic is contained in West Africa—that we're not saying goodbye to Ebola in North America. We need to protect ourselves. The evidence suggests simple things can make a difference.

We each need to adopt the focus of "Ebola-Aware Living."

CHAPTER FOUR

Following Basic Hygienic Practices

In the world of infectious diseases a key concept is that of an "infective dose." This refers to how many germs are needed to cause clinical infection. Although this varies from person to person based on immune system health and other factors, generalities can be made for different infectious illnesses.

For example, one of the most common causes of food poisoning in America, *Campylobacter jejuni*, sickens some two million of us annually. However, it takes exposure to between 500 and 10,000 bacteria to cause infection. The more serious and rarer food-borne illness, typhoid fever, requires in the range of 15-1000 *Salmonella typhi* bacteria to cause symptomatic illness. However, when it comes to Ebola, non-human primate research suggests as few as one to ten *aerosolized* organisms can be infective.

The latter figure may sound dismal. Nonetheless, here is the important point: Less exposure is always better. Although some might fault me for the analogy, limited exposure to viral proteins is at the heart of vaccine therapy. I'm not suggesting anyone try to get "just a touch of Ebola exposure"—perhaps an organism or two—in an attempt to render himself immune. (If that is your greatest concern, at least two groups are making promising strides toward a human

Ebola vaccine, aspects of which were nicely summarized by Thomas Burton in his recent *Wall Street Journal* article.)

What I am saying is this: Some of us may be exposed to the Ebola virus. If we are, the smaller the magnitude of that exposure, the better. In this chapter, I'll review some simple practices that can decrease our risk of contracting the illness, even if exposed.

Oh, yes, one more thing. Even if you never come face to face with Ebola, the strategies in this chapter will decrease your risk of a host of diseases that are actually statistically more likely to kill you than even Ebola. Don't misunderstand me—I'm not talking case-fatality rate (the number of people who have clinical illness compared to the number who die). I'm talking death in absolute numbers.

For example, only a small portion of those who contract influenza die from it. However, each year during the U.S flu season, thousands lose their lives from this infectious disease and its complications. Since influenza strains vary in severity, a "good year" may see in the range of 3,000 deaths, with a "severe year" claiming up to 50,000 lives. Hygienic practices may well help you prevent this less-glamorous killer.

Hand Washing

At the foundation of infection control is good hand washing. Most illnesses are either transmitted by contact with mucous membranes (such as those associated with your eyes and nose) or by ingesting the infectious agent.

One of the most effective ways to transmit a host of diseases, from Ebola to the common cold to the flu, is by simply rubbing your nose or eyes with contaminated hands. That's right, if the Ebola virus is on your hands, simply contacting those moist body tissues can, in effect, inoculate you with the virus.

The message is simple: Wash your hands before touching your face—especially your eyes or nose. (We'll come to your mouth shortly.) If you can't get to tap water, use an alcohol-based cleansing solution. Many expert groups suggest that these sanitizers must contain at least 60 percent alcohol to be effective in eliminating Ebola.

I'm talking here about routine from-here-on-out lifestyle practices. One point I've been trying to emphasize is this: If Ebola infection rates ramp up on U.S. soil, we may receive low-grade exposures without ever being aware of the source. Scrupulous hygiene practices can make a significant difference in low-grade exposure scenarios.

Hand Washing 101

Everyone knows how to wash their hands, right? Dead wrong. Just hang out in a busy public restroom for a while, and you'll quickly realize most people either don't have a clue—or behave as if they don't. Common mistakes include the following:

▶ **Too short a time.** Effective hand washing requires twenty seconds of scrubbing with soap and water (warm or cold).

▶ **Turning a water faucet off with your washed hands.** Once you have washed, whether you are at home or in a public restroom, don't touch the faucet with your clean hands. The ideal scenario involves using the paper towel you dried with to turn off the water.

▶ **Assuming a paper towel dispenser lever is clean.** If you are in a public restroom, wash your hands, then depress the paper towel lever. Wash again before taking the paper towel. Use the paper towel you dried with to release more toweling if you need it—or to save the next person from washing twice as you just did.

▶ **Opening the bathroom door with your now-washed hands.** Doorknobs are high-risk surfaces. Use a paper towel to open the door—or you'll likely contaminate your hands on the way out.

Sounds like a pain, eh? Well, honestly, I follow these practices myself on a regular basis. Are you now ready to tell me to get a life? Actually, these practices are a very small inconvenience when you merely calculate the saving of missed days from work due to colds and flu—even if Ebola were not in the picture.

I witnessed a practical illustration of this some years ago when a co-worker learned about these hand-washing strategies. He put them into practice. Soon afterward, he excitedly told me how he had already noticed substantially fewer viral illnesses.

Decreasing Your Risk of Oral Ebola Exposure

Most infectious illnesses are either transmitted via mucous membranes or by ingestion but not both routes. Unfortunately, Ebola can be transmitted effectively by either.

This brings hand-washing again front and center. By all means, don't eat or put your hands in your mouth for any reason without washing them first (or at least using hand sanitizer with a minimum 60 percent alcohol content).

When it comes to eating, your choice of foods also makes a difference. A number of cases of Ebola have been traced to the eating of "bushmeats." This does not necessarily mean bats, one of the putative reservoirs for Ebola. It can also include other carnivorous animals. For example, we have already seen that dogs can be infected with Ebola. Of course, in some parts of the world, this common American pet is used for human consumption. An Ebola-infected hound could be your own ticket to Ebola. And "vegetarian" animals are not necessarily safe. Although many non-human primates like chimps and gorillas are thought to be mainly plant eaters, eating their flesh has been linked to Ebola outbreaks.

Neil Nedley, MD, a popular author on mental health subjects, made a fascinating observation during a recent academic presentation. He pointed out that no cases of Ebola have ever been linked to the ingestion of animals deemed "clean" by the ancient Mosaic health laws. (If curious to know which creatures were so designated, check out Leviticus, chapter 11, in a modern translation of the Bible.)

Applying Public Health Code in Your Own Home?

As far as I know, every state public health department mandates that patrons of self-service buffets or restaurants must obtain a clean plate before taking "seconds."

Because as many as 67 percent of those with acute Ebola infection have the virus in their saliva, this ubiquitous public health practice takes on greater significance in homes and other informal meal settings. You see, if someone has been eating off his plate, then puts additional food on that same plate, the potential exists for the serving dish to be contaminated. The classic scenario occurs when the individual touches the serving utensil to his dirty plate.

Think about the chain of events that could occur at one of those popular community "bean suppers" in New England. Richard, a Caucasian, recently back from a business trip to West Africa, raises no suspicions. (He's not wearing a T shirt that says "I survived my recent trip to Guinea," nor is he making small talk about his recent travel.) However, he not only has been exposed to Ebola but has actually been incubating the disease—and, unknown to him or anyone else, is destined to be diagnosed with Ebola the following day. Richard's saliva is already contaminated with infectious particles which unavoidably find their way onto his spoon as he eats. The viruses then become intermixed with the beans in his bowl.

When Holly invites him to try some of the beans she has prepared, Richard doesn't hesitate to walk back over to the serving table. As he dishes out her beans, they stick to the serving spoon, so he taps it on the side of his own bowl. Thus, the Ebola virus finds its way to the serving spoon. Of course, Richard puts that spoon back in the serving dish. Things have now come full circle. The virus is now in Holly's dish, waiting for the next unsuspecting human to dig in.

Another far-fetched scenario? Perhaps. But perhaps not. Remember, investigations of other Ebola outbreaks in Africa have left experts and lay people alike wondering about the source of exposure for certain people. Personally, I think contaminated food, hands, and fomites (those inanimate objects we talked about earlier) are more likely to be the sources rather than aerosolized, airborne Ebola.

But even if there's never an Ebola-infected Richard in your community, let me tell you one of the fringe benefits of hygienic food serving. Evidence indicates such practices can decrease your risk of stomach ulcers. That's right. A common cause of what are called peptic ulcers is a germ known as *Helicobacter pylori*. *H. pylori* can also be transmitted by oral-to-oral transmission, the very type of transfer we illustrated at that New England "potluck."

Just a bit much to swallow at your dining room table? Then do this at a minimum. If you must serve yourself on a plate from which you have already eaten, ensure that the serving utensils never touch your plate. Just make it a family rule. If someone slips up, simply get a clean serving utensil rather than putting the contaminated one back into the serving dish.

Avoiding Other Exposures

One of the more sobering aspects of the Ebola virus is just how long someone can harbor the virus in his or her body—even after recovering from infection. In a review of all Ebola studies to date, viral persistence following symptom onset was found to vary by body fluid:

- Skin (sweat?): 6 days
- Saliva: 8 days
- Breast milk: 15 days
- Blood: 21 days
- Eye (tears): 22 days
- Urine: 23 days
- Rectal secretions (stool?): 29 days
- Vaginal secretions: 33 days
- Semen: 101 days

Although it is possible some of these body fluids have the virus in such low concentrations as to be an unlikely source of transmission, the infective dose of Ebola is so small that we shouldn't take chances. For example, although semen consistently reveals the greatest Ebola virus persistence, sexual transmission of Ebola has never been proven. Nonetheless, the related Marburg virus can be sexually acquired.

For me the conclusion is simple: Even if you are monogamous, when Ebola is present in a region, engage only in protected sex. If your partner has recovered from Ebola, I would follow such recommendations for at least three months.

Remember too, some individuals can have inapparent infections. When someone has such a low-grade, asymptomatic infection, we would expect their viral loads to be magnitudes lower than someone with an active clinical infection. However, there still is the remote possibility that infection could be transmitted to an unwitting sexual contact. I recommend erring on the side of caution.

Healthcare Workers

Although the Centers for Disease Control may have been criticized for some of their early responses (or lack thereof), they have a very solid track record in the public health community. From my vantage point, the CDC continues to generate solid recommendations that have adjusted for earlier oversights. As the current outbreak plays out, new observations may reveal other areas for fine tuning. However, I see no compelling need to try to improve on their current guidelines for health professionals caring for Ebola patients.

Having said that, I will make one vital point. If you are a healthcare worker, and based on the best information available (including the insights found in this book), don't feel you are being offered appropriate protective gear or other controls for a given situation—you should not silently acquiesce. Before entering into a situation you are not convinced is safe, I would recommend you insist on one of two things. Either your employer provide you with that which you believe you need, or provide you with evidence to help you realize you are being overscrupulous in your concerns. No one should be required to go into a high-risk situation unless he or she is convinced that every reasonable step has been taken to minimize chances of personal harm.

Summary

When Ebola virus is present in an area, even individuals who never get clinically ill can harbor the virus. For this reason, caution is warranted—we need to be *Ebola Aware*—and not only in high-risk settings. Practice good hygiene when it comes to hand washing, food preparation, and food serving, and you stand to significantly decrease your risk of ever contracting the disease.

CHAPTER FIVE

Other Strategies Following Ebola Exposure (or Potential Exposure): An Overview

Amentor during my Internal Medicine training hammered down one of medicine's most important aphorisms: "The first step in treatment is diagnosis." Perhaps nothing is more critical to remember when discussing Ebola infection.

As has been effectively communicated by the lay press, once someone has sustained a known, significant Ebola exposure, he or she should follow indicated quarantine protocols. The level of quarantine may depend on how high-risk the exposure is deemed by public health personnel. Although quarantine protocols are typically coupled with rigorous, regular screening, any exposed individual should be especially vigilant regarding the development of early symptoms of clinical Ebola infection.

Early diagnosis is critical. Although there is currently no specific approved therapy for Ebola infection, prompt diagnosis puts a patient and his caregivers in the best position to benefit from both experimental and established therapies. Among the latter are what we call in medical circles "supportive measures." Although far from glamorous, these practices can be lifesaving.

As eloquently expressed in the title of a recent *New England Journal of Medicine* article penned by Dr. François Lamontagne and his collaborators, we can do "Today's Work Superbly Well" by "Treating Ebola with Current Tools." The gist of the article is that one of the main advantages derived from treating Ebola in a Western hospital is the availability of standard "supportive measures," such as providing intravenous fluids. You don't need a medical degree to realize that a person with the severe gastrointestinal symptoms that often accompany florid Ebola infection (think vomiting and diarrhea) can rapidly experience depleted fluid stores. In this setting a patient can rapidly deteriorate.

The *New England Journal* authors, all of whom have apparently dealt on the front lines of Ebola infection in West Africa, remind us of Ebola's typical course: "After a few days [of clinical illness]… the predominant clinical syndrome is a severe gastrointestinal illness with vomiting and diarrhea. Volume depletion with a range of metabolic disorders ensues, and hypovolemic shock ultimately occurs." In plain English, these experts remind us that the path that leads to many Ebola-related fatalities is something called "hypovolemic shock"— blood pressure so low that vital organs cannot get adequate, life-sustaining circulation.

The emphasis of these front-line Ebola experts is truly eloquent in its simplicity. They bemoan their observation that many of the West Africans afflicted with Ebola do not get simple, basic supportive care. Giving intravenous fluids and correcting deficits in sodium and potassium that typically occur with diarrhea and vomiting can truly transfer a patient from the wards of death to the halls of life. And those IV fluid needs may be enormous. It is not uncommon for an Ebola patient to require five to ten liters daily. (Think in the range of one to three *gallons*, not pints.)

But what's true in West Africa is true here as well. If the

Ebola crisis worsens on American soil, you or a loved one may find yourself not only with clinical illness but also in the hands of an inexperienced healthcare team. (Granted, this book is calculated to decrease that possibility—but no matter how preventive minded we are, the possibility exists that a serious exposure could lead to full-blown Ebola illness.)

If the unthinkable happens, and you or a loved one is hospitalized for Ebola in an institution unfamiliar with Ebola treatment, don't let the professionals become sidetracked trying to secure the latest experimental drugs. Getting the most cutting-edge agents is fine in itself—but not if it causes the team to lose sight of tried-and-true remedies. Advocate for careful attention to the basics—appropriate I.V. fluids and careful monitoring of electrolytes such as sodium and potassium.

Enter New Drugs

Don't misunderstand me. If I'm stricken with Ebola and my condition is deteriorating in spite of my clinicians doing "superbly well" in providing supportive care, put me on the list for experimental therapies. The most promising therapies fall into two categories:

▸ **Antibodies Against Ebola.** The most old-school concept has been illustrated by Dr. Kent Brantley's willingness to donate his own blood or serum to Ebola sufferers. As an Ebola survivor, the doctor's blood has a liberal supply of antibodies against the rogue virus. Theoretically, so long as another patient has a compatible blood type, an infusion of his serum could provide a potent immune system boost.

Before sharing his own blood, Brantley—while in the throes of Ebola—was himself the recipient of the same low-tech antibody therapy when he received blood from one of his young patients, an Ebola survivor. Additionally, Dr. Brantley was given cutting-edge, high-tech antibody therapy in the form of the experimental drug, ZMapp. That agent is a genetically engineered ("monoclonal antibody") mix of three different antibodies, all targeting components of the Ebola virus.

▸ **Antiviral Drugs.** Among the most promising of these are brincidofovir, which has shown anti-Ebola activity in laboratory studies, and TKM-Ebola. The latter is designed to undermine Ebola's ability to self-replicate. It has already shown promise in non-human primate studies.

Still other therapies are under investigation for what is called post-exposure prophylaxis—approaches designed to lessen the risk of disease when someone has just experienced a significant exposure. Health professionals would benefit from an excellent review of this topic written by Mike Bray, MD, MPH, available from the subscription medical service, *UpToDate.* Bray's bottom line recommendation provides solid counsel for lay people and health professionals alike: "In the event of an exposure, filovirus experts should be contacted for advice about the status of experimental therapies. In the United States, such consultation can be obtained by contacting the Special Pathogens Branch at the Centers for Disease Control and Prevention (CDC)."

More Post-exposure Prophylaxis

Although a healthcare professional may well be aware of an Ebola exposure in the course of caring for an infected patient, lay people may not have any indication of lower grade exposures that could occur in the context of more widespread Ebola activity in North America. This realization argues again for all of us adopting an *Ebola-Aware Lifestyle*—before the epidemic further heats up.

With this in mind, we now move on to seven vital aspects of such a lifestyle:

1. Adequate Hydration
2. Regular Physical Exercise
3. Optimal Nutrition
4. Adequate Sleep and Rest
5. Smoking Cessation
6. Stress Management
7. Social Support

CHAPTER SIX

Adequate Hydration

As we have already seen, the term *prophylaxis* refers to preventive practices. Since Ebola can present with severe gastrointestinal symptoms, it seems prudent (following a known exposure to Ebola or merely residing in a region where Ebola is potentially circulating) to ensure adequate hydration on a daily basis. Some may question the importance of staying "tanked up" fluid-wise, when you are following other aspects of an *Ebola-Aware Lifestyle*. However, we have already noted that one of the quickest routes to Ebola-induced death involves fluid and electrolyte imbalances. I'm not suggesting that good hydration will obviate the need for I.V. fluids if Ebola strikes. Nonetheless, if you experience vomiting and diarrhea as early symptoms, being well hydrated provides a margin of safety while seeking to obtain definitive medical care.

Bigger Reasons for Adequate Hydration

This book's greatest purpose isn't helping you survive clinical Ebola illness—although I believe the strategies recommended can aid you in the setting of such a serious infection. My foremost goal is to help you avoid ever facing clinical Ebola infection. With this end in mind, adequate hydration is critical.

Among the most common symptoms of dehydration are an increase in fatigue and a corresponding decrease in mental vigor. Even mild levels of dehydration can be accompanied by a lack of mental clarity. In a now-classic study conducted by French researchers, Cian and colleagues, seven healthy men were exposed to a variety of conditions. When the subjects became dehydrated either by exercise or by heat exposure, their mental performance deteriorated, as documented by psychological testing. Cognitive abilities including perceptive discrimination and short-term memory all suffered. Fatigue increased.

In another scientific publication, St. Louis University researchers Wilson and Morley summarized dehydration's impact in one of the more vulnerable segments of the population: "Dehydration in older adults has been shown to be a reliable predictor of increasing frailty, progressive deterioration in cognitive function and an overall reduction in quality of life."

Why Is This Important?

Because I'm recommending a lifestyle—an *Ebola Aware Lifestyle*—anything that affects your brain and your resolve are serious matters. Let's imagine you're a health professional, caring for a hospitalized Ebola patient. If you've been getting enough sleep but have lost your mental edge due to poor hydration, you're already putting yourself at risk. One popularized overseas Ebola case occurred when a health professional was taking off her personal protective garb. Before completing the routine, she unthinkingly rubbed her eye with a soiled glove. A relatively short time later, she was an Ebola casualty.

We can all see the stakes are extremely high when dealing with an overtly ill patient with extremely high Ebola virus loads. However, I've been trying to make the case that healthy lifestyle practices can dramatically decrease our risk of infection in situations where we may face much smaller exposures. We need to keep cognitively astute to follow a lifestyle that maximally decreases infectious disease risk.

Beyond Ebola

One of my most popular lay lecture series is entitled "The Methuselah Factor: Longevity Plus" (available in DVD format on my website, www.compasshealth.net). The entire two-hour mini-series is devoted to the health benefits of optimizing blood fluidity, to which optimal hydration is key. I won't take time here to share research on how keeping well hydrated—and following other blood-fluidity enhancing strategies—can pay huge dividends in terms of decreasing your risk of stroke, diabetic complications, and even cancer. However, let me just briefly mention an amazing study that emphasizes the far-reaching benefits of water drinking. Even if you never come anywhere close to a single Ebola virion, adequate hydration could well be lifesaving.

Over a decade ago, Dr. Jacqueline Chan and fellow researchers at Loma Linda University made a remarkable discovery. They found a simple practice could make the difference between dying from a heart attack and avoiding such a fate. That practice was merely drinking more water. We're not talking about copious volumes of that most available of all beverages. When compared to those drinking less than two glasses of water daily, women who drank more than five glasses per day cut their risk of a fatal heart attack by 41 percent. Men received an even greater benefit, registering a 54 percent risk reduction.

What About Other Beverages?

Perhaps as startling as the benefits of water drinking in the Loma Linda research were the effects of other fluids. Chan's team found that other beverages, looked at collectively, had the opposite effect. Men who drank more than five glasses of other fluids per day were 46 percent *more* likely to die from a heart attack than those who consumed other beverages less than twice daily. Women who more frequently downed other beverages experienced an astonishing 147 percent increase in fatal heart attack risk!

I know what many of you are wondering. Surely, not every other beverage is harmful. Probably not. But two of America's favorites are surely not our friends—at least when we return to an assessment of beverages in the light of infectious diseases such as Ebola.

Alcohol and Immunity

His was a very sad case. Albert may have seemed "up in years" when I met him as an Internal Medicine resident. However, from the vantage point of my now more mature life, he was really quite young—in his mid-60s, as I recall. Nonetheless, in that hospital room decades ago, he seemed to be at death's door. His rapid spiral was occasioned by an infectious illness. No, not Ebola, but pneumonia. Despite our best efforts, it seemed nothing our medical team could do would reverse Albert's inexorable death spiral. All too soon, he breathed his last.

In reflecting on his demise years ago, one factor stood out in all our minds: Albert's heavy use of alcohol. We were convinced even then, that if he had not had so much alcohol on board, his immune system could likely have held its own—at least with some support on the medical end with antibiotics and other necessary interventions. You see, in large doses there is absolutely no question that one of the world's most popular beverages is immunosuppressive.

When it comes to an *Ebola-Aware Lifestyle*, there is little question. All heavy drinking is out. No more bingeing. Cross drunkenness off the list.

But what about "moderate drinking"—how does *that* impact immune health? If you were to wade through the medical literature, you would likely be confused. Some studies raise concern; others seem to assuage fears.

Without going into great detail, let me give you my distillation of the research: Alcohol in any amount is immunosuppressive. However, because every alcoholic beverage is made from plant products, none of those beverages are pure ethanol. They all retain some plant chemicals or phytochemicals, many of which have salutary properties. As we'll see in an ensuing chapter, many phytochemicals have immune-enhancing properties. For this reason, when consumed in small or "moderate" amounts, alcoholic beverages may not seem to undermine immune function.

If you've been reading between the lines, you may already see the danger of those appearances. Why not just have some unfermented grape juice rather than wine? Why not bypass the juice altogether and simply opt for table grapes? These other strategies will give you the immune-enhancing benefits of the phytochemicals without neutralizing those benefits with immunosuppressive alcohol. Think about it. If you are really determined to do all you can to decrease your risk of infectious diseases, why not follow the optimal program?

OK. I can hear some of you already. If your favorite beverage is not going to cause your immune system to tank, you're still planning to have some anyway. Besides, some of you might be reasoning, if a surface reading of the medical literature isn't decisive, why should you trust me more than any other "moderate drinking" medical advocate?

Here's why: In looking at cumulative immune system impact, one of our best indicators is cancer risk. If cancer cases increase with a certain practice, we should suspect either the presence of cancer-inducing substances or immune-suppressing agents—if not both. In the case of moderate drinking, there is no uncertainty. Take note of the results from one of the world's largest prospective studies, The European Prospective Investigation Into Cancer and Nutrition (EPIC). Their research, involving over 300,000 participants, squares with many other studies. Any amount of alcohol consumption measurably increases cancer risk.

Is Caffeine Safe?

Do you really want the answer? Remember, at the end of the day, my job in this book is to give you an optimal immune-enhancing lifestyle program. If you are exposed to Ebola, you want "all hands on deck" when it comes to your immune system. However, I'll grant you this: None of us are likely to follow perfectly every aspect of this program every day of our lives.

Confession: I'm working on a tight deadline with this book and I'm not getting an optimal amount of sleep. (You'll find in a future chapter that this too is unbalancing to the immune system. So I'm hoping I don't come in contact with the Ebola virus in the near future.) However, back to the issue on hand. I'm not drinking caffeine to remain more vigilant. Why?

We've known for years that caffeine stacks the deck against your immune system. As detailed in the well-documented "Wake up and smell the coffee: Caffeine, coffee, and the medical consequences," author T. Chou described how caffeine ramps up stress hormone levels. I'll spare you all the physiology, which brings in such esoteric concepts as antagonism of adenosine receptors and alterations in cellular concentrations of cyclic adenosine monophosphate. The bottom line you already knew: Caffeine is a stimulant. But what most lay people don't realize is that stimulation comes from ramping up stress hormones such as cortisol.

Cortisol and related "glucocorticoids" are anti-inflammatory steroids that have immune-suppressive effects. Such compounds may seem desirable if you have tendonitis, inflammatory bowel disease, a flare of rheumatoid arthritis, or even a significant asthmatic tendency. In these autoimmune and inflammatory conditions, inflammation may seem more of an enemy than a friend. However, when it comes to infectious diseases such as Ebola, your immune system is your biggest ally. And ramping up your cortisol levels—whether by caffeine or through other means—will impair your defenses.

But What About the Cognitive Benefits?

I made a case for staying hydrated to keep mentally astute. If you're dragging, couldn't caffeine be a good thing cognitively? Not exactly. The great Russian scientist, Pavlov, reportedly dubbed caffeine, "bad habit glue." In other words, if you're serious about the premise of this book; namely, that a prudent lifestyle may spell the difference between contracting or not contracting clinical Ebola infection, then you'll think twice before ingesting a substance that may make it difficult to embrace healthier behaviors.

Interested in a concrete example? In 2000 we published a summary of our work with nicotine addiction in *Complementary Health Practice Review*. There, we documented that, after some four to six months of follow-up, none of those who went through our residential stop smoking program returned to tobacco if they also refrained from coffee. Among those who didn't heed our advice to remain caffeine-free, a significant number returned to their nicotine addiction.

Consequently, if you're trying to make significant lifestyle changes in light of Ebola awareness, this doctor recommends removing caffeine from your program.

Summary

Do you want to stay cognitively sharp and give your immune system an edge? Drink plenty of water. Don't settle for caffeinated or alcoholic beverages.

CHAPTER SEVEN

Regular Physical Exercise

R egular, moderate, exercise is a boon to the immune system. As such, it plays a vital role in keeping our immune system functioning optimally. I have not been able to find any research specifically assessing the impact of exercise or fitness on clinical Ebola infection risk. However, our knowledge of other human-virus interactions suggests there may well be a relationship. After all, many researchers have documented benefits of regular, moderate exercise in helping our immune systems ward off viral invaders.

For example, Dr. David Nieman and colleagues at Appalachian State University documented significant antiviral benefits accruing from regular physical activity during the fall and winter cold and flu season. In their study of more than 1,000 men and women (ranging in age from 18 to 85), they found that those who engaged in regular aerobic activity (five or more days per week) had 43 percent fewer respiratory infections than those who were predominantly sedentary (exercising less than twice weekly).

Most people realize that "aerobic" exercise refers to more than indoor "dance aerobics." However, I still find many patients who are confused by the term. Simply put, any activity that gets you breathing harder, raises your heart rate, and involves large muscle groups such as your arms or legs is aerobic. This would include walking, riding a bicycle, jogging, and playing tennis, as well as indoor group exercises to music. These "whole body" exercises seem to afford immune enhancement.

Of further interest, Nieman's team found that benefits accrued not only from being more active but also from actually being more fit. (Sure, you'd expect these to go together, but they are different. Activity looks at behavior; fitness looks at the results of those behaviors.) The researchers noted a similar virus-preventive effect when subjects were stratified based on their fitness levels. Those in the upper third of fitness had 46 percent fewer days experiencing cold and flu symptoms than the least fit third.

Because of the demonstrated anti-viral effects of consistent moderate exercise and fitness, I include daily physical activity as an integral part of an *Ebola-Aware Lifestyle.* Having said this, I can anticipate the response of many readers. After all, in some thirty years of medical practice I have seen the eyes of many a patient glaze over when I recommend regular physical activity.

However, we're really not talking about some onerous burden. Some years ago I was reviewing the exercise literature with a very definite purpose in mind. I was searching for *the* study that showed how *little* exercise one could get and still receive measurable benefit. Because thousands upon thousands of studies have been conducted on this topic, there was little likelihood I could review *all* of the exercise literature. However, I found research documenting that *as little as six minutes* of moderate activity could measurably improve one's immune system.

Here's the take-home message. Make a daily commitment to physical activity. No excuses. Really, I've heard them all.

(Of course, if you have health concerns about the safety of a particular type of activity, by all means check with your doctor first.)

Think about it. You make time every day to eat and sleep; why couldn't you make exercise just another "given"? And if you honestly think you don't have time in your day to squeeze in six minutes, please contact me. You'll be the first person to ever tell me that with a straight face.

Two Caveats

First, I'm not saying that six minutes is the optimal duration of activity for immune system benefit. So long as you are not overdoing it, thirty minutes or more is probably much better. In fact, I generally recommend my patients work up to accumulating at least sixty minutes of exercise daily. This is especially true if they are overweight. Because carrying excess pounds has immune-disrupting effects, even modest amounts of weight loss (typically aided by physical activity) can be immune enhancing.

Second, if some exercise is good, more is not necessarily better—especially if you push yourself to exhaustion. The research is equally clear when it comes to the benefits of moderate exercise and the immune-suppressing effects of intense or exhaustive exercise.

Consider the work of Australian researcher M.W. Kakanis and his collaborators, as published in a 2010 issue of *Exercise Immunology Review.* Using ten elite male cyclists as their test subjects, they detailed the impact of extreme exercise (two hours of intense bicycling) on immune function. The Australian team documented a number of findings that were of serious concern. One of the most important when it comes to Ebola was this: a progressive fall in Natural Killer cells (a particular class of enemy-destroying white blood cell). This trend began with the onset of exercise and continued during and after exercise, until Natural Killer (NK) cell concentrations had dropped by some 40 percent four hours after the athletes had finished cycling. This magnitude of depression persisted for another four hours. Even twenty-four hours later, NK cell function had not returned to normal. This is extremely worrisome in light of Ebola concerns, since NK cells play a key role in the body's defenses against this pathogen.

If you're not an athlete, can you dismiss all such concerns regarding over-exercise? No. Some years ago, Dr. Harold Mayer and I collaborated with other investigators to look at the effects of exercise on sedentary individuals. One of the interesting—yet intuitively obvious—observations that emerged was this: What may look like moderate exercise for a fit person is often extreme exhaustive exercise for the unfit. We showed in our study that sedentary individuals actually did better in terms of weight loss and body fat reduction if they combined short periods of rest with their exercise. I would not be surprised if their more moderate approach to exercise had also yielded better immune results. But, alas, we made no such measurements.

Summary

If you are serious about an *Ebola-Aware Lifestyle*, exercise will be a part of your daily routine. Listen to your body. Don't overdo. Even take breaks if necessary. And remember, as little as six minutes of moderate activity can yield measurable immune system benefits.

CHAPTER EIGHT

Optimal Nutrition

Nearly two decades ago, Kaiser Permanente physician Steve Provonsha published a fascinating paper. His review of the medical literature corroborated his own clinical findings. Namely, when humans consume animal tissue (red meat, poultry, etc.) the body is duped into thinking its own tissues are compromised, triggering a stress response. Provonsha reasoned that the similarity of animal products to human tissue (once touted as a reason to eat these "complete protein" sources) was anything but health-giving. Of concern to us, Dr. Provonsha found that the stress hormone cortisol was ramped up by the consumption of animal foods. His focus was on the deleterious connections between cortisol, other stress hormones, and diabetes. Nonetheless, we have observed that this same compound can also impair our immune systems.

If we are serious about living an *Ebola-Aware Lifestyle*, Dr. Provonsha's work encourages us to curtail our intake of animal products. In fact, a number of lines of evidence suggest that a vegetarian diet is best calculated to enhance immune function.

Fruits and Vegetables to the Rescue

If you are looking at ways to obtain the highest quality nutrition on a per calorie basis, you will spend a lot of time shopping in the produce section. The vitamins and minerals found in abundance in plant foods offer significant promise for decreasing our risk of viral illness. Although we don't yet know how much this applies to Ebola, we have enough evidence to encourage at least two things in our quest to limit the ravages of the current epidemic.

▸ First, we should all ensure a liberal intake of plant foods.

▸ Second, optimal blood levels of vitamins and essential minerals should be prioritized.

Consider some of the evidence. For many years researchers have noted connections between nutritional deficiency and either increased susceptibility to infectious diseases or more severe disease if infection occurs. One classic example is provided by the anti-viral properties of the vitamin A family. Population research (epidemiology) has revealed that children deficient in vitamin A are at greater risk of severe measles infection. In such situations, administration of high-dose vitamin A supplements can shorten the duration and severity of this viral illness.

Observations such as these leave me convinced that if we want to decrease the impact of Ebola worldwide, we must think beyond both conventional therapies (such as fluid and electrolyte management) and high-tech solutions (such as monoclonal antibodies and other investigational drugs). Granted, an effective Ebola vaccine would be perhaps the most wonderful of all advances. However, in the meantime, I believe we should never lose our focus on the importance of nutrition.

This topic provides ground for fertile research. Do those who die from Ebola tend to have lower levels of vitamin A or other nutrients? Ebola exposures being equal, do individuals with clinical illness tend to have poorer nutritional status than those who develop inapparent infections? Although we don't currently know the answers to these questions, fascinating evidence is emerging.

Earlier this year, German researcher Andreas J. Kesel and colleagues published amazing data on a vitamin A–derived compound called Retinazone (RTZ). This agent has been shown to have powerful effects against viruses as diverse as Hepatitis C, HIV, and, yes, even Zaire-type Ebola. Before rushing out to the nearest drug store and supplementing your diet with vitamin A, let me warn you. I have never recommended vitamin A supplements to any American patient (most all of us tend to have adequate levels). Vitamin A can be toxic. Among its toxicities is immune system compromise.

The safer member of the vitamin A family, when ingested in foods, is beta-carotene. You cannot get Vitamin A toxicity from this plant source of the vitamin. However, high doses in supplement form may still have immune-weakening effects.

Although I've spent time at length speaking about the vitamin A family, we could well have spent our energies speaking about other antioxidant vitamins (such as C and E) or essential minerals like selenium and zinc. These and other essential nutrients may all play a role in ensuring optimal immune function.

Here's how I synthesize the data on nutrition and Ebola risk reduction in the face of potential infectious exposures: Eat a variety of nutrient-rich fruits, vegetables, whole grains, nuts, and seeds.

Additional Benefits From Plant Foods

When we looked at alcoholic beverages in chapter 6, I alluded to the health-enhancing effects of phytochemicals. There, I made the case for eating more plant foods (rather than imbibing fermented beverages) in order to best reap their benefits. An emphasis on phytochemicals is again warranted at this juncture.

A simple definition is first in order. Phytochemicals are natural plant compounds that are *not* essential for life (i.e., not vitamins or essential minerals), yet can exert a variety of beneficial human health effects. In other words, by ramping up plant sources of nutrition, whether they be fruits, vegetables, whole grains, nuts, or seeds, we maximize our phytochemical intake.

The Ebola-prevention connection here is simple. Many of these phytochemicals have beneficial effects on the immune system, either through dampening inappropriate inflammatory responses or through other mechanisms. On top of all this, you reap derivative benefits, since a variety of phytochemicals have been shown to aid in cancer prevention, eye health preservation, cartilage repair, hypertension treatment, and dementia prevention.

Plant-strong diets have also been shown to aid in weight reduction. For example, vegans (who eat only plant foods) tend to be at significantly lower body weight than those who eat more animal products. As alluded to in the previous chapter, carrying extra weight is an immune system liability.

Finally, when it comes to Ebola, there's at least one other reason to think seriously about eating lower on the food chain (more plants—less meat, milk, eggs, and cheese). This was graphically illustrated during my own travels to West Africa some years ago. On a number of occasions, the rural village where I was staying was enveloped in a thick cloud of smoke. I learned there were a number of contributors to the poor air quality, but one caught me by surprise. Some of the villagers would burn swaths of forest to flush out rodents that they would then kill for food. Their consumption of bushmeat was being driven by a very real need to have adequate calories to survive.

Consuming less of the world's food resources doesn't guarantee there will be more food for starving Africans (any more than cleaning my plate as a child helped the malnourished masses). However, if we eat more plant foods, we are clearly leaving a smaller footprint on our planet. Theoretically, the five or ten pounds of grain that it may take to create a pound of animal protein could feed me as well as a number of others—especially if we could address political and distribution problems. This is not just idle musing. If we could remove the incentive for Africans to eat unclean jungle meats, we might do more to reduce the worldwide risk of Ebola than just about anything else.

Caveats

Eating more fruits and vegetables is a healthy practice for *most* people, with some rare exceptions. For example, if you have kidney failure, compounds such as potassium and magnesium can build up to dangerous levels in your body. Since these minerals are found in abundance in plant products, the red flag immediately goes up.

Certain medications may put you at risk from dramatic dietary changes. A case in point is provided by some high blood pressure medications which cause potassium retention. Again, ramping up fruit and veggie intake may get you into trouble if you are taking such drugs.

Like any of the advice in this book, make sure you check things out with your health care provider—especially if you have significant illness or are taking prescription medications.

Vitamin D and Immunity

In order to make this an easily digestible volume, I've tried to limit my discussion of vitamins to the example of Vitamin A. However, my conscience will not allow me to omit at least a brief mention of Vitamin D. This "sunshine" vitamin can be a particular problem in darker races—even in sun-drenched equatorial Africa. What is so remarkable about vitamin D are its profound immune system effects, as well as its frequent deficiency. It would be fascinating and perhaps therapeutically revolutionary to check blood levels of 25-OH vitamin D (the compound accurately reflecting body vitamin D stores) in those suffering from Ebola. I would not be at all surprised if merely improving vitamin D status would make some impact in decreasing the risk of acquiring and/or succumbing to Ebola infection.

When it comes to an *Ebola-Aware Lifestyle,* I believe we must all ensure that we are not vitamin D deficient. If you don't know where you currently stand, I would recommend having your own 25-OH vitamin D level checked. If it is low, work with your doctor to start on supplementation right away. If Ebola visits your community or the plane you're on, you may be glad you did.

CHAPTER NINE

The Four S's (Sleep, Smoking Cessation, Stress Management, and Social Support)

When it comes to an *Ebola-Aware Lifestyle,* there are other immune-enhancing and health-promoting practices besides the pillars of hydration, diet, and exercise. In this chapter we look at four that elude many in our ranks. Each is calculated to help us maintain a fit immune system and consequently, the upper hand in any Ebola conflict.

Rest and Sleep

Perhaps one of America's strangest "values" is the ability to apparently "get by on little sleep." So enamored was I at these prospects that, as a busy college student, I consistently shorted myself on sleep. I thought I was doing just fine—or, to be honest, pretty well. However, I didn't realize I was displaying tell-tale signs of sleep deprivation. One of those was short sleep latency. Falling asleep "when your head hits the pillow" is not a great talent—it's the result of insufficient rest.

Despite our national obsession with getting by with less, *more sleep* is what our immune systems really need. Adequate sleep is vital to the production of restorative compounds such as melatonin, growth hormone, and interleukin 1 (IL-1), all of which either help our bodies broadly or enhance immune function specifically.

While sleep deprivation causes helpful immunostimulatory compounds to be downregulated, other pro-inflammatory agents are ramped up. Michael Irwin, MD, and colleagues from the Semel Institute for Neuroscience at UCLA elegantly documented this in a 2006 *Archives of Internal Medicine* report. The scientists recruited thirty healthy volunteers and compared their immune systems on four hours of sleep (3 A.M. to 7 A.M.) with nights when they were better rested (sleeping from 11 P.M. to 7 A.M.). Irwin's team found that sleep deprivation turned on the genes that make inflammation-stimulating compounds such as Interleukin-6 (IL-6) and Tumor Necrosis Factor-alpha (TNF-α). The immune-unbalancing effects were profound, as IL-6 production was ramped up more than three-fold, while TNF-α essentially doubled.

In the face of sleep deprivation, this perfect storm of muting the good and amplifying the bad further imbalances our immune systems and leaves us less able to fight infectious invaders as mundane as the common cold or as frightening as Ebola.

Indeed, in 2009, Sheldon Cohen, PhD, and his colleagues brought these discussions back into the world of practical virology. Over a period of four years Cohen's team recruited 153 healthy volunteers (men and women between the ages of 21 and 55). Each reported their sleep duration and sleep efficiency (percentage of time in bed actually sleeping) for two full weeks. After documenting their sleep habits, the researchers gave each subject nasal drops containing rhinovirus-39, a "common cold" virus. I'll spare you the details of the elegant controls that Cohen's team implemented to ensure that any symptoms were indeed due to those nasal drops (quarantine for five days; pretesting of nasal lining to exclude incubating viral illness, etc.). Clearly, the study design left one impressed that what the researchers wanted to measure was indeed being measured.

So what did they find? Those who slept less than seven hours per night were roughly three times more likely to come down with a cold than those getting more than eight hours nightly. Those with intermediate amounts (seven to eight hours per night) had a 63 percent increased risk compared to the longest sleepers. Striking relationships were also logged when it came to sleep efficiency. Spend more time in bed awake, and your risk for the common cold rises.

Of course, it would be highly unethical to repeat the same experiment with Ebola virus. But I wonder if the results would be similar. Isn't it interesting to think that many of those exposed to Ebola are in sleep-deprived situations of caring for a loved one or (in the case of African health professionals) a whole ward of desperately ill patients? It's sobering to think that if we could just ensure more sleep for Ebola caregivers, we might be able to decrease the toll from the disease.

There's another message here, of course. If you find it easy to fall into one of my bad habits; namely, overworking prior to a long trip with the expectation of crashing on the plane, it may be time for us both to think seriously about changing that practice. With Ebola in circulation, it doesn't strike me as a particularly good idea to enter those close quarters sleep deprived and consequently, immune imbalanced.

If you're among the ranks who feel that dialogue such as this unnecessarily ramps up the fear factor when it comes to Ebola, just read the work of brain scientists discussing the results of sleep deprivation—with Ebola totally out of the equation. If you want to read something frightening, now we're talking.

To dive into a predigested discussion on the topic, check out Alice Park's well-researched "The Power of Sleep." You'll read there of the very real concerns that our short sleeping habits are a form of lifestyle Russian roulette, dramatically increasing our risks of neurodegenerative diseases such as Alzheimer's.

If you haven't yet picked up the refrain, an *Ebola-Aware Lifestyle* just plain makes sense, even if Ebola is soon deported from North America, never to return.

Rather than fear-mongering, I see my role as echoing Ebola's wakeup call. Let's get serious about healthier living—including getting more sleep.

Smoking Cessation

Few people in the Western world do not recognize, at least to some extent, the enormous health toll exacted by cigarette smoking. After all, it is hard for the world's leading cause of preventable disease and death to escape notice. Even among those held firmly in the addictive tentacles of nicotine, few will debate the causal connections between smoking, lung cancer, emphysema, and heart disease. However, the immune-suppressing effects of smoking are not as broadly appreciated.

When I first began helping patients stop smoking in the 1980s and 1990s, researchers had isolated more than 3,000 chemicals from tobacco smoke. Today, that figure is upward of 7,000. Those staggering numbers reflect more than compounds innately in tobacco. A significant cadre of chemicals—including some of the most dangerous ones—are formed from pyrolysis (burning).

Among those 7,000 chemicals are four classes of agents that destine many smokers to cancer. They include carcinogens (compounds capable of causing cancer themselves), co-carcinogens (compounds that can cause cancer when working in conjunction with other agents), tumor promoters, and tumor accelerators. Still other tobacco smoke chemicals derange the immune system. Some of that derangement results in the immune system attacking the very organs and tissues it is supposed to protect. The destruction of elastic tissue in the lungs, for example, feeds the insidious process of emphysema.

If you were waiting for another reason to stop smoking, here it is: If you want your immune system functioning optimally, you need to call it quits.

Remember, although the risk of aerosolized Ebola virus has been downplayed, there are data suggesting just such spread may have occurred in the past. While we pray that Ebola will be quickly contained in the Americas and never surface again, the scope of the West African epidemic suggests we are not yet finished with this pathogen. As we prepare for the possibility of greater exposures to come, let's ensure that our lungs are in the best shape to meet any potential challenges.

Stress Management

By now we've talked enough about the stress hormone *cortisol* that it has become a very familiar compound—if it wasn't already. Having traced cortisol's immune-reducing properties in conjunction with issues as diverse as caffeine consumption, overweight, and sleep deprivation, there's no need to belabor the obvious. Simply put: Stressful situations ramp up hormones that degrade immune functioning.

For decades researchers have demonstrated that things as seemingly innocuous as watching a stressful video film (now doesn't that date the studies?) to giving a speech in public (one of the most stressful scenarios for thousands) to taking an exam can cause measureable immune impairment. The dots have also been connected when it comes to viral illness. Stressed individuals are simply more susceptible.

So what are we to do about all this? Doesn't it seem unfair

that many of us are getting stressed out about Ebola at the very time we need to control stress better in order to have the best chance of evading clinical illness at this foreigner's hands?

In reflecting on this irony, I thought about my recent chance encounter with a physician mentioned earlier in this book, Neil Nedley, MD. Dr. Nedley is known to many for his comprehensive natural approaches to mental health issues such as stress and depression. His community-based classes have been convened across the globe.

What was percolating in my mind was Nedley's remark that Ebola's grasp would never have been so firm had all West Africans followed the Mosaic principles of eating (as recorded in the Bible's Leviticus 11). The stress-management connection finally gelled. What Dr. Nedley was saying was simply this: There are remedies for the Ebola epidemic that grow out of his spiritual worldview. From interviews of Dr. Brantley, I imagine he would likely say the same, particularly since he credits his life to divine intervention as well as medical heroics.

Here's where I am going with all of this: Connect with your own spiritual roots. That heritage may be very different than that of Drs. Nedley or Brantley, but within it may lie the greatest stress management keys in coming to grips with Ebola's menacing face.

Social Support

If you've been tempted to cancel flights, reschedule a cross-country train trip, or even hold off on shopping during peak times, you're not alone. Fear of communicable disease can definitely impact our social connectedness. However, before withdrawing into your own cocoon, consider this. Social support is one of the most powerful aids to our immune systems.

One of my favorite illustrations of this medical truth is drawn from the huge Nurses' Health Study conducted by Harvard University. The research team—which has been following over 100,000 nurses since 1976—published a fascinating study in a 2006 issue of the *Journal of Clinical Oncology*. Lead author Candyce H. Kroenke and colleagues identified 2,835 women from the Nurses' Health Study who were diagnosed with stage 1 to 4 breast cancer between 1992 and 2002. But they did more than collect standard medical data about those women. The investigators also assessed the level of social support each was receiving in both 1992 and 2000. When they analyzed the data, they found something remarkable. When compared with nurses who were well integrated socially, those who were socially isolated had more than double the risk of dying from breast cancer during the course of the study. Additionally, the socially isolated women were 66 percent more likely to die from any cause.

Here's how the investigators made sense of their observations: "Social-emotional support, often provided by a confidant, may reduce stress and hypothalmus-pituitary-adrenal–axis reactivity, which might improve immunosurveillance against cancer recurrence." In plain English, they were saying that the stress system, which ultimately involves your adrenal glands (and you guessed it—they're the source of cortisol production) can be toned down by social support. Keeping cortisol levels low is good for your immune system. It's good for cancer. And it's good for Ebola. Staying socially connected aids you on all these fronts.

Summary

A host of simple things can go a long way toward helping us evade Ebola. Getting enough sleep, avoiding smoking, controlling stress, and staying socially connected may all help make the difference between an immune system that can resist an Ebola challenge and one that will succumb to it. And as I opined earlier, most of these values are not all that different than those espoused by your grandmother or many of the world's great spiritual traditions.

CHAPTER TEN

Conclusions

I hope you agree with me. We need to change the dialogue. We've been so focused as a nation on the "invading of Ebola" that we've lost sight of our privilege of "evading Ebola."

Let me back up. I'm very thankful for the efforts of the CDC and NIH, as well as the US military. By the way, their commitment to make a difference in West Africa is truly extraordinary. Kudos.

In spite of some bumps along the way, other government branches have been admirably rising to the occasion. But after reading this book, don't you see the glaring problem with our national mentality? As a people we've been looking at Ebola as a rogue enemy against whom we are largely helpless. We've been behaving as if our only recourse is a dramatic federal government rescue—and when that hasn't happened on our time schedule, our angst has been palpable.

However, if we realize the significance of the "inapparent infection" phenomenon, the whole dialogue changes. It is likely that thousands of Africa's denizens have been visited by Ebola and never so much as fallen ill.

Rather than reassuring ourselves that it is impossible to come in contact with the virus from contaminated food, aerosolized secretions, or inanimate objects, let's own up to the truth. Evidence suggests the possibility of Ebola exposure from any of those sources—as unlikely as each might be.

This is not a call to fear but a call to empowerment. It is not a call to decrease the quality of our lives by hiding in our bedrooms in Hazmat suits but rather to embrace the healthiest lifestyle possible—an *Ebola-Aware Lifestyle.*

At the end of the day, my recommendations to evade Ebola are in reality an invitation to live a life that decreases our risk of *all* the world's greatest killers and cripplers, from heart disease to cancer to dementia.

Let's make a commitment together to evade Ebola.

Appendix

Reality has a way of getting one's attention. Within twenty-four hours I'll begin a series of flights as I crisscross the country recording radio shows and giving lectures. As I think of the prospect of flying through some of our nation's busiest airports I have to ask: What happens if one of those "Matilda" scenarios evolves? Have I communicated in this book everything I myself would do if I had a significant Ebola exposure?

I'll be honest. There's one thing I've neglected to share that would definitely be on my list of post-exposure prophylaxis. I've refrained because it's the most theoretical of all my recommendations. However, since I believe it could make a significant difference, I'll at least mention it so you can add it to your list of options: Hyperthermia treatment (also known as fever therapy).

You might be wondering why I would recommend treating with fever an infection that causes fever. I'll explain in a moment. However, first let me provide a little background.

My appreciation for fever therapy dates back probably more than thirty years when, as a medical student, I first read a book on natural therapies authored by the physician team of Calvin and Agatha Thrash. As part of their rationale for hyperthermia (artificially raising the body temperature) they reviewed the history of syphilis treatment. The Thrashes recounted how, before the advent of antibiotics, various means were used to induce fever in an attempt to treat advanced syphilis that had spread to the nervous system. They related how a 1949 medical journal reported that a good percentage of cures were effected "in those patients who were treated early and were conscientious enough to complete the full course of treatment."

Natural practitioners for decades have used similar methods to try to treat stubborn infectious illnesses. The rationale is simple: Within reasonable limits fever is helpful. It speeds up the immune system's function and may give it the upper hand in dealing with infection.

For this reason, fever in illness is generally beneficial, unless the temperature goes too high. The situation with Ebola is more complicated. By the time someone develops a fever, it generally indicates their immune system lost the initial battles, and the virus has now commandeered immune functions. In this scenario, uncontrolled fever may present a serious threat.

Here's my question: What happens if I started giving myself fever treatments right after exposure to Ebola? Might this help my immune system get the upper hand? I don't know the answer, but I think it is worthy of consideration.

How to Give a Fever Treatment

I wouldn't presume in these pages to tell you how to do so, for no one should administer such a treatment on himself. You should ideally have an ally in a health professional who would deem that it did not present any undue risk. Then at least initially, a healthcare worker would administer and observe the treatment. This is not to say a family member could not ultimately render such therapy—but they should not do so at first.

Once you have a serious Ebola exposure, you should be quarantined. But before being exposed, if you want to get information—or even personal instruction on the fever therapy intervention—I would recommend one of three health care facilities:

▶ Uchee Pines Institute in Seale, Alabama (near Columbus, GA); www.ucheepines.org

▶ Weimar Institute in Weimar, CA (between Sacramento and Lake Tahoe) at www.newstart.com

▶ Wildwood Lifestyle Center and Hospital in Wildwood, Georgia (just outside of Chattanooga, TN); www.wildwoodhealth.org

Do You Want More Help on Actually Implementing an *Ebola-Aware Lifestyle*?

Even after reading the material in this book, you may still feel you want more individualized instruction on how to implement an *Ebola-Aware Lifestyle*. You may also want to benefit from social support, having others help you on such a healing journey. If so, I can unequivocally recommend the three centers above. They not only have experience administering hyperthermia treatments, they also can give you a comprehensive, individualized program focused on immune enhancement.

Remember, however, that such intensive education is for individuals before they have a known Ebola exposure. Once exposed, you should avoid travel and follow recommended quarantine precautions.

What if You Don't Live Anywhere Near Those Select Facilities?

Other programs are available that likely have similar expertise. However, those just mentioned are the only three centers for which I can personally vouch. Nonetheless, there are other community-based (and even online) curricula that cover all the elements of my Ebola-Aware Lifestyle—barring perhaps hyperthermia. Here are the ones I recommend:

▶ The Complete Health Improvement Program—developed by Preventive Medicine pioneer, Dr. Hans Diehl. www.chiphealth.com.

▶ CREATION Health—developed by one of the world's largest health systems, Florida Hospital based in Orlando, FL. www.creationhealth.com.

▶ The Nedley Depression and Anxiety Recovery Program (a holistic program that targets more than merely mental health)—developed by Dr. Neil Nedley (mentioned earlier in this book). www.nedleydepressionrecovery.com.

One Final Story and an Additional Resource

This book was written on very short notice to address a public health emergency that had stepped onto American soil. When I was searching for an editor for this work, I believe I was providentially directed to Ken McFarland. McFarland is not only an experienced editor but a fellow-author on the topic of Ebola. Of perhaps even greater practical interest, he runs a news aggregator devoted exclusively to Ebola. If you want to keep on top of this rapidly evolving topic, put his website on your daily read list: www.ebolanewsupdates.com.

Selected References

Chapter 1

Baize, S; Leroy, EM; Georges-Courbot, MC; et al. "Defective humoral responses and extensive intravascular apoptosis are associated with fatal outcome in Ebola virus-infected patients." *Nat Med.* 1999; 5:1-5.

Leroy, EM; Baize, S; Volchkov, VE; et al. "Human asymptomatic Ebola infection and strong inflammatory response." *Lancet.* 2000. Jun 24;355(9222):2210-5.

Chapter 2

Allela, L; Boury, O; Pouillot, R; et al. "Ebola virus antibody prevalence in dogs and human risk." *Emerg Infect Dis.* 2005. Mar;11(3):385-390.

Centers for Disease Control and Prevention (CDC). Ebola Virus Disease. Accessed 20 October 2014 at http://www.cdc.gov/vhf/ebola/index.html.

Centers for Disease Control and Prevention (CDC). Review of Human-to-Human Transmission of Ebola Virus. October 17, 2014. Accessed 19 October 2014 at http://www.cdc.gov/vhf/ebola/transmission/human-transmission.html.

Wauquier, N; Becquart, P; Padilla, C; et al. "Human fatal zaire ebola virus infection is associated with an aberrant innate immunity and with massive lymphocyte apoptosis." *PLoS Negl Trop Dis*. 2010. Oct 5;4(10).

World Health Organization. "Ebola haemorrhagic fever in Zaire, 1976." *Bulletin of the WHO*, 56(2):271-293, 1978.

Chapter 3

Busico, KM; Marshall, KL; Ksiazek, TG; et al. "Prevalence of IgG antibodies to Ebola virus in individuals during an Ebola outbreak, Democratic Republic of the Congo, 1995." *J Infect Dis*. 1999. Feb;179 Suppl. 1:S102-107.

The Centers for Disease Control and Prevention (CDC). Ebola virus disease Information for Clinicians in U.S. Healthcare Settings. October 15, 2014. Accessed 20 October 2014 at http://www.cdc.gov/vhf/ebola/hcp/clinician-information-us-healthcare-settings.html.

DeRose, DJ; Charles-Marcel, ZL; McLane, GL; Blum, DC; "Vegan-Based Lifestyle for Diabetic Neuropathy: A Model for Managed Care" presented at the American Public Health Association's 126th Annual Meeting; Washington, D.C. November 1998.

Chapter 4

Burton, TM. "Why the Work of Dr. Nancy J. Sullivan Could Be Key to a Potential Ebola Vaccine." *The Wall Street Journal* (Online). Oct. 19, 2014. Accessed 20 October 2014 at http://online.wsj.com/articles/ebola-vaccine-push-ramps-up-1413762856.

Centers for Disease Control and Prevention (CDC). Review of Human-to-Human Transmission of Ebola Virus. October 17, 2014. Accessed 19 October 2014 at http://www.cdc.gov/vhf/ebola/transmission/human-transmission.html.

Centers for Disease Control and Prevention (CDC). Wash Your Hands. December 11, 2013. Accessed 20 October 2014 at http://www.cdc.gov/Features/HandWashing.

Food and Drug Administration (FDA). *"Salmonella* species" and *"Campylobacter* species" in *Bad Bug Book: Foodborne Pathogenic Microorganisms and Natural Toxins Handbook.* 2012. Accessed 20 October 2014 at: http://www. fda.gov/downloads/Food/Food-borneIllnessContaminants/ UCM297627.pdf.Public Health Agency of Canada. Ebolavirus. August 2014. Accessed 20 October 2014 at: http://www. phac-aspc.gc.ca/lab-bio/res/psds-ftss/ebola-eng.php.

Chapter 5

Bray, M. "Diagnosis and treatment of Ebola and Marburg virus disease." *UpToDate.* Oct 20, 2014. Accessed 21 October 2014 at http://www.uptodate.com/contents/diagnosis-and-treatment-of-ebola-and-marburg-virus-disease#H8.

Lamontagne, F; Clément, C; Fletcher, T; et al. "Doing Today's Work Superbly Well—Treating Ebola with Current Tools." *N Engl J Med.* 2014, Sep 24. [Epub ahead of print].

Chapter 6

Chan, J; Knutsen, SF; Blix, GG; Lee, JW; Fraser, GE. "Water, other fluids, and fatal coronary heart disease: the Adventist Health Study." *Am J Epidemiol.* 2002, May 1;155(9):827-833.

Chou, T. "Wake up and smell the coffee. Caffeine, coffee, and the medical consequences." *West J Med.* 1992. Nov;157(5):544-553.

Cian, C; Barraud, PA; Melin, B; Raphel, C. "Effects of fluid ingestion on cognitive function after heat stress or exercise-induced dehydration." *Int J Psychophysiol.* 2001, Nov;42(3):243-251.

DeRose, DJ; Braman, MA; Charles-Marcel, ZL; et al. "Alternative and complementary therapies for nicotine addiction." *Complementary Health Practice Review*. 2000, Fall; 6(1):98.

Lovallo, WR; Whitsett, TL; al'Absi, M; et al. "Caffeine stimulation of cortisol secretion across the waking hours in relation to caffeine intake levels." *Psychosom Med*. 2005, Sep-Oct;67(5):734-739.

Schütze, M; Boeing, H; Pischon, T; et al. "Alcohol attributable burden of incidence of cancer in eight European countries based on results from prospective cohort study." *BMJ*. 2011, Apr 7;342.

Wilson, MM; Morley, JE. "Impaired cognitive function and mental performance in mild dehydration." *Eur J Clin Nutr*. 2003, Dec;57 Suppl 2:S24-29.

Chapter 7

DeRose, DJ; Mayer, HC; Charles-Marcel, ZL; et al. "Intermittent training aerobic exercise, the thyroid, and weight loss." *Obesity Research*. 2000, Oct; 8(S1): 82S.

Kakanis, MW; Peake, J; Brenu, EW; et al. "The open window of susceptibility to infection after acute exercise in healthy young male elite athletes." *Exerc Immunol Rev*. 2010;16:119-137.

Nieman, DC; Henson, DA; Austin, MD; Sha, W. "Upper respiratory tract infection is reduced in physically fit and active adults." *Br J Sports Med*. 2011, Sep;45(12):987-992.

Warfield, KL; Perkins, JG; Swenson, DL; et al. "Role of natural killer cells in innate protection against lethal ebola virus infection." *J Exp Med*. 2004, Jul 19;200(2):169-179. Epub 2004 Jul 12.

Chapter 8

Benson, S; Arck, PC; Tan, S; et al. "Effects of obesity on neuroendocrine, cardiovascular, and immune cell responses to acute psychosocial stress in premenopausal women." *Psychoneuroendocrinology.* 2009, Feb;34(2):181-189.

Gröber, U; Spitz, J; Reichrath, J; et al. "Vitamin D: Update 2013: From rickets prophylaxis to general preventive healthcare." *Dermato-Endocrinology.* 2013, Jun 1;5(3):331-347.

Kesel, AJ; Huang, Z; Murray, MG; et al. "Retinazone inhibits certain blood-borne human viruses including Ebola virus Zaire." *Antivir Chem Chemother.* 2014, Apr 11;23(5):197-215.

National Institutes of Health. Office of Dietary Supplements. Vitamin A Fact Sheet for Consumers. June 05, 2013. Accessed 22 October at http://ods.od.nih.gov/factsheets/VitaminA-Consumer/.

Provonsha, S; Wade, C; Sherma, A. "Syndrome-AC: non-insulin-dependent diabetes mellitus and the anabolic/catabolic paradox." *Med Hypotheses.* 1998, Nov;51(5):429-438.

Slavin, JL; Lloyd, B. "Health benefits of fruits and vegetables." *Adv Nutr.* 2012, Jul 1;3(4):506-516.

Chapter 9

American Lung Association. Stop Smoking. 2014. Accessed 22 October 2014 at http://www.lung.org/stop-smoking/about-smoking/health-effects/smoking.html.

Arcavi, L; Benowitz, NL. "Cigarette smoking and infection." *Arch Intern Med.* 2004, Nov 8;164(20):2206-2216.

Brown, R; Price, RJ; et al. "Interleukin-1 beta and muramyl dipeptide can prevent decreased antibody response associated with sleep deprivation." *Brain Behav Immun.* 1989, Dec;3(4):320-330.

Cohen, S; Doyle, WJ; Alper, CM; et al. "Sleep habits and susceptibility to the common cold." *Arch Intern Med.* 2009, Jan 12;169(1):62-67.

Irwin, MR; Wang, M; Campomayor, CO; et al. "Sleep deprivation and activation of morning levels of cellular and genomic markers of inflammation." *Arch Intern Med.* 2006, Sep 18;166(16):1756-1762.

Kroenke, CH; Kubzansky, LD; Schernhammer, ES; et al. "Social networks, social support, and survival after breast cancer diagnosis." *J Clin Oncol.* 2006, Mar 1;24(7):1105-1111.

Mehta, H; Nazzal, K; Sadikot, RT. "Cigarette smoking and innate immunity." *Inflamm Res.* 2008, Nov;57(11):497-503.

Park, A. "The Power of Sleep." *Time Magazine.* 22 Sept 2014. 184(11):5258.

Appendix

Thrash, A; Thrash, C; *Home Remedies: Hydrotherapy, Massage, Charcoal, and Other Simple Treatments.* Uchee Pines Institute. 1981.

For More Information

If you enjoyed Dr. DeRose's *Evading Ebola,* you'll love his other resources. At his www.compasshealth.net website you'll find free materials as well as opportunities to purchase his popular DVD health education programs. (And if you're still struggling with the prospects of making some of the lifestyle changes Dr. DeRose recommends, pick up a copy of his motivational mini-series, *Changing Bad Habits for Good,* at http://www.compasshealth.net/purchase/).

Keep on Learning!

Now that you've enjoyed Dr. DeRose's information-rich best-selling new book—*Evading Ebola*—consider continuing to learn from some of his best seminars in DVD form on the following pages.

Reversing Hypertension Naturally

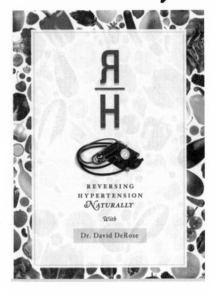

JOIN DR. DAVID DeROSE in this three-part series as he helps you understand the dangers of high blood pressure and then provides strategies to help you control or even reverse it naturally!

Price: $26.95 + $5 S & H

Order online at:
http://www.compasshealth.net/purchase/

Reversing Diabetes Naturally

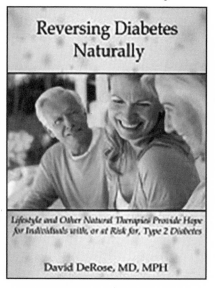

THIS LIFE-CHANGING SERIES unlocks the power of a non-drug approach for type 2 diabetes. Viewers will learn how to address the root cause of this disorder known as "insulin resistance" and much, much more. (Four presentations, approximately 1-hour each; i.e., approx. 4 hours total run time.)

Price: $40 + $5 S & H

Order online at:
http://www.compasshealth.net/purchase/

The Methuselah Factor: Longevity Plus

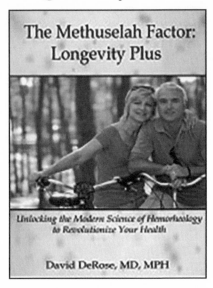

IN THIS DVD SERIES, Dr. DeRose unlocks the fascinating science of hemorheology, showing how we can increase our likelihood of living longer and better by following simple lifestyle practices that enhance blood fluidity. (Two presentations, approximately 60-min each; i.e., approx. 2 hours total run time.)

Price: $20 + $5 S&H

Order online at:
http://www.compasshealth.net/purchase/

Listening to the Buffalo

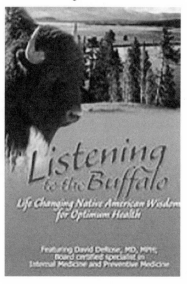

STARTING WITH THE TRUE STORY of an American Indian-raised homesteader who survived a buffalo stampede, Dr. DeRose takes a scientific look at the Native Americans who held bison in high esteem. You'll gain amazing insights into how modern science validates simple lifestyle strategies that can help prevent or treat diabetes and other lifestyle-related metabolic conditions. (Two presentations, approximately 30-min each; i.e., approx. 1 hour total run time.)

Price: $20 + $5 S&H

Order online at:
http://www.compasshealth.net/purchase/

Changing Bad Habits for Good

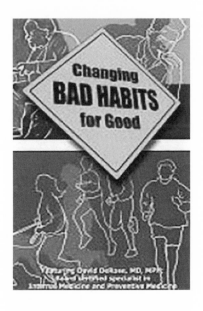

IF YOU KNOW WHAT YOU should be doing for your health but are having trouble translating that into practice, this DVD is for you. Finally master the dynamics of health behavior change in an engaging, practical way. You'll learn to develop new enjoyments, enjoying high quality living at the same time you shed unwanted habits. (Two presentations, approximately 30-min each; i.e., approx. 1 hour total run time.)

Price: $20 + $5 S&H

Order online at:
http://www.compasshealth.net/purchase/